Kultivating Kids!

*Garden Therapy
That Helps ALL Kids*

Kultivating Kids!

*Garden Therapy
That Helps ALL Kids*

by Debbie Kissel & Lu Luby

*Published by
Bulls-Eye Creative*

Produced by
Bulls-Eye Creative
a division of
Bulls-Eye Promotions, Inc.
P.O. Box 390123
Snellville, GA 30039
www.bulls-eye.net

Written by Debbie Kissel and Lu Luby
Art Direction: Toro Luby
Custom Illustrations: Cory A. Luby

Printed in the United States

Second Edition
ISBN: 0-9771849-3-5
(previous ISBN 0-9771849-0-5)

Table of Contents

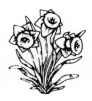

Forward

I have never had much of a "green thumb"; however, I have had the experience of appreciating the tranquility and healing that a garden has to offer. Amidst the activity and stress that our daily lives can impose upon us, a garden can offer a place to be ourselves and to regain our balance. I have had the fortune of working with children with special needs and raising my own 4 children. I have seen the tremendous impact that a sensory environment, particularly, a sensory garden can provide both to special needs and to those who consider themselves without special needs. This guide is a cookbook to creating a sensory garden for any population in nearly any location. It is laid out so clearly and easy to follow that even someone such as myself will find it a true assistance in creating that very special place. I applaud both Debbie and Lu who have put their time, energy and hearts into making this guide a reality in hopes that it will assist you and your special needs individuals. It is in our gardens where we really come to know ourselves and where we find hope.

Ilana M. Danneman, PT

Introduction

I love kids!

I adore gardens!

And, don't you think the two would be a perfect match?!

In most cases, the answer is a definite and resounding "Yes!" Almost all kids are attracted to the immense sensory pleasure and wonderment of Mother Nature's bountiful garden. From mud pies, collecting worms, jumping in leaves, riding in a wheelbarrow, getting dirty, watching things grow, and digging...the array of beauty and sensation in nature absolutely captivates most children. As they enjoy the garden, they develop new skills, have fun, play, and develop self-confidence.

Some of the things children learn in the garden include:
- **Responsibility**- from caring for and tending plants, and being a 'helper'
- **Understanding**- as they learn cause and effect, like watching plants struggle without water
- **Self confidence**-by taking on responsibility, especially when growing food that can be eaten
- **Love of nature**-learning about the sensations of the outdoors in a safe and beautiful place
- **Reasoning and discovery**-of simple construction, botany, science, art and nutrition
- **Interpersonal skills**-communicating and cooperating to work as a team

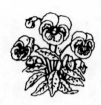

This is actually a small part of what a child leaves the garden with. Since play is such an important part of learning it is always great to give the child time and space for self-discovery. How heavy to fill a bucket of water? How hard to push on a wheelbarrow? What can be put in a wagon? Because as much as a child learns about the outside world, they are also learning about what their bodies can do.

Some of the skills kids develop in the garden can include:
- **Body awareness**-an internal sense of where their bodies are in space when performing activities
- **Using both sides of the body**-for pulling, pushing, raking, digging and sweeping
- **Hand preference**-as a preferred hand becomes more and more skilled with repetitive jobs
- **Motor planning**-such as thinking of what the body can do, planning, and then executing that garden task
- **Balance**-being stable while carrying, lifting, and loading objects. Navigating the change in terrain
- **Coordination**-from digging a straight line, to planting beans by hand
- **Ocular tracking**-from scanning for birds and butterflies to finding acorns

Most children are naturally attracted to the garden and it takes no effort to get them there...and keep them engaged. Some of the children I love, however, can't make sense of their senses. They have **Sensory Processing Disorder (SPD)**. SPD is to the brain what indigestion is to the stomach. Information from the senses gets jumbled, lost, or processed incorrectly. Typical areas of poor integration

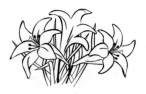

include touch, muscles and joints, and the movement system. These kids with SPD, often have poor attention spans, hyperactivity or low energy, difficulty being touched, and coordination issues, Faced with sensory challenges, these kids can sometimes come across as tense, or unhappy.

In the garden a sensory avoider may:
- Not want to get dirty
- Refuse to interact with wet textures
- Dislike the feel of grass, especially on their feet
- Fatigue when digging
- Become irritable in the warm/cold extremes
- Complain of certain smells "stinking"
- Wipe their hands frequently
- Say "I'm falling" when walking on slight hills
- Have no interest in tasting grown vegetables or fruit

Some children with SPD may be an under-responder to sensory input and in the garden may:
- Not notice how dirty they are or that their nose is running
- Be unaware that their tools are knocking down other plants
- Not notice a change of temperature and keep a sweater on if it is hot
- Not engage in touching or exploring things that most kids enjoy
- Show no awareness if injured

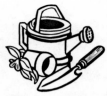

Those children that are sensory-seekers in the garden may:
- Enjoy the messy process so much, they forget the task at hand
- Need to touch and feel everything in sight
- Constantly fidget
- Refuse to keep their shoes on
- "Dive" into the activities
- Bump or touch other children

For myself, I consider being in the garden 'work therapy.' I enjoy the outdoors and doing heavy work. 'Work therapy' gives all of my muscles a workout. I tend to breathe deeply. I feel rejuvenated and relaxed. For kids with SPD, the garden offers the opportunity to do "heavy work." The input to the muscles and joints helps to calm the child's system, allowing the sensory information to process more normally. The opportunities to push, pull, lift, bend, dig, rake, and sweep are abundant. The opportunities to "cultivate" whole kids...not just gardens, is abundant, too.

One of the authors of *Kultivating Kids*, Debbie Kissel, is passionate about helping kids with Sensory Processing Disorder. Her experience and nurturing ability can be found throughout the creative hands-on activities suggested in the book. With decades of experience in early childhood, her sensitivity to those struggling to process sensory input is extraordinary. No matter where Debbie is, that is where the children flock. She gives permission to every child, to enjoy being the unique individuals that they are.

Debbie's co-author, Lu Luby is just as passionate about all children being able and capable. An avid gardener herself, Lu is an artist in many medias. The garden rooms she creates are artistic, uplifting, and always contain a special place for children. Her palate of plants, contains the most sensory rich experiences whether in color, scent, sound, or texture. There is also something pragmatic in the way Lu's garden designs incorporate raised beds, wheelchair accessible paths, and multi-sensory plant material in the most important places. Add a touch of whimsy, a splash of magic and you'll be captivated by how easy it is to replicate one of Lu's plans for gardens for all children, particularly those with sensory or physical impairments.

My favorite thing about *Kultivating Kids* is that the authors never forget that the real richness in gardening are the experiences that help the KIDS grow and evolve. The gardens in this book have produced beautiful bouquets, fun craft projects, and even some edible vegetables, but it is the bushels and bushels of laughter and fun that has cultivated the children most of all.

Suzanne Wilkinson
Occupational Therapist

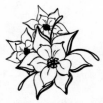

Gardening: the Sensory Experience

Wouldn't it be wonderful to create a place to explore and experience using only one's sense of sight, sound, smell, touch or taste? A place where one can relax, unwind and discover gentle sounds, new fragrances, bursts of color and textures never imagined in the classroom or home?

This is what a Sensory Garden can be. Too often, Nature at her best is overlooked as a teacher, caretaker or therapist. Simple gardening can offer a host of pleasant experiences that will reach our senses in a variety of ways. Can you feel the warmth of a puddle of water that has been heated by the sun as you scoop it from a copper container? Or finding a quiet nook surrounded by beautiful greenery and flowers of all colors? Then, while admiring the sight, hearing the soothing music of wind chimes? The mind, body and spirit are all touched by even the simple texture of bark or taste of a sprig of fresh mint.

Many feel that gardening is for those with a talent or a green thumb, but using a variety of plans and recommend plants and accessories, anyone can make a peaceful, beautiful area for all to enjoy - especially children with varying abilities. Most children love to dig in the dirt, plant, water and pick flowers and vegetables.

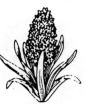

Children find a garden a place that gives them a sense of peace and grounding. This includes children with varying abilities. Learning takes place, senses are aroused and an appreciation of the world around us develops. Gardens can be simply planted to allow for wheelchairs or those walking with assistance, offering a unique, open-air classroom. This book contains information to help plan and source any size garden, on any budget and in any planting zone. The information will also help in choosing plants and materials that will appeal to all five senses.

Sensory Gardening can help improve mind, body and spirit. Using thinking skills, memory and observation touches the mind. The physical benefits include increased muscle tone and range of motion by using muscles differently as one tends to a plant. And the spirit...the spirit soars as it sees new life and growth.

Groups for whom gardening as therapy have proven successful include not only the abled bodied population, but developmentally disabled, physically challenged, recovering substance abusers and others. By tending plants, those involved experience a hands on connection with nature and the life cycle. A sense of excitement and anticipation are often felt as they wait to see what happens next. Researchers at the University of Florida have found that just walking through a beautiful sensory garden lowers stress levels. Participating in gardening isn't the only way to reduce stress. The sensory experience of the colors, scents and sounds helps one appreciate the peace a garden provides.

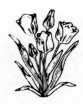

Our Five Senses

Gardening affects all our senses. Most of us are more sensitive than we realize. Our sensory experience build neurological pathways in the brain and reinforce existing ones.

Our Sense of Sight

Take a moment, close your eyes and visually see the plants in the garden. Are they all green? Are they all the same size? Are they all the same shape? What else is there? Is the garden just flowers, trees and bushes? Adding a simple water feature brings the calming affect of water. A few colorful kites or flags add more color to attract our eye. Attracting birds and butterflies contributes to the beauty of the garden, (See the section on Birds and Butterflies later in this book for more information). A water source other than a hose can add another dimension to the beauty of the garden. A copper whirling watering tool is just as easy as a plain old hose and even more functional! The wonderful sight of a garden delights our sense of sight just by the variety that is always present.

The plants you choose should offer variety. Easy to care for perennials return year after year and may be a good choice to start with. Choosing plants according to their mature size will help in your planning and that information is included here for you.

What about water? Solar fountains are very popular, economical and safer than a pond or large fountain. These fountains provide the beauty of water in the garden and appeal to other senses as well. Allowing the water to spray gently across the body or to dipping the hands into the fountain as it streams down is peaceful and relaxing.

Our Sense of Sound

Now, what do you hear in your garden? Listen to the rustle of leaves, grass, birds and water? Add a wind chime to gently provide music that soothes the soul. Sound is an essential element of a comfortable atmosphere.

Our Sense of Smell

Take a deep breath. Can you smell the soil? Is the fragrance of fresh flowers reaching your senses? Plants that have various scents are included here to help you maximize your garden's own personal scent. Rich, healthy soil not only smells good, but your plants thrive in it. Even water has its own scent. Studies have shown that scent provides memories and lasting impressions. Strong scents such as pine, sage or cedar produce clean and enjoyable scents. It is natural for us to smell flowers. Encourage children to also smell the leaves, the soil, the water and more.

Our Sense of Touch

Have you seen a plant that begs to be touched? Lamb's ear? Fuzzy plumes of pampas grass? This garden is for touching. But be careful - no thorny roses here! Included in this book are lists of plants recommend because of their texture, color and of course, safety. Your garden can be the most touchable around! Encourage children to feel the smooth rocks, the bumpy barks on the trees or in your mulch, the water - cooled or warmed by the sun. How about a sensory fence? Imagine a small two-inch or larger fence made of different textures of wood or willow that children can feel as well as provide a barrier in your garden! You can spend a day just touching and identifying textures!

Our Sense of Taste
What about taste? Sure, you can eat vegetables grown in your garden, but what plants can you eat? Mint, lemon balm, dill, violet leaves and stems (not your houseplant variety) are all safe.

Our Sixth Sense
Though not an official "sense," what about that feeling inside yourself? Intuition is so basic and hard to define. Making your garden a comfort zone that encourages interaction will enable that sense to feel good — to feel welcomed. In this comfort zone, the world opens anew. Take time to enjoy nature. Don't just stop and smell the flowers — EXPERIENCE them and all that is in your garden!

Sensory gardens provide children an understanding of the impact that nature has on all of their senses. Do children enjoy gardens and truly appreciate them? Of course they can! Gardening opens another door to learning, feeling and experiencing responsibility - a sense of hope as plants grow and change.

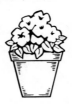

Fun Things to do with Kids in the Garden

Make Mud

Allow the kids to add water to good dirt a little at a time. Encourage them to mix it with their hands to a nice thick consistency. Pour some in a basin or straight onto the ground and encourage them to put their bare feet in the mud, squishing between their toes.

It's easy to clean up — just rinse away! The wonderful warmth if done in the heat of the day — or the coolness if in the shade or with cool water - of the mud is a very nice, relaxing feeling!

Weaving

Weave dried grasses, large slender leaves and yarn. These can be used as little seats in the garden, liners in plant trays and pieces of art. The textures of the various elements appeal to many children.

Make Flower and Leaf Prints

Dip flowers, leaves, grass or anything else in your garden in tempera paint. Press on paper.

Make a Worm Bin

Buy or build a plywood box (great project for a dad or a Boy Scout) approximately three feet by two feet wide and one foot high. Fill the bin to almost the top with shredded newspaper, dead leaves or shredded cardboard. Add a couple of handfuls of dirt and slightly moisten the contents. Then mix and add worms. Redworms are highly recommended; just ask any bait and tackle shop or gardening center for a handful.

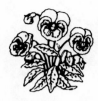

What do worms eat? They love fruits and vegetables or anything organic. They don't like meat, junk food, cake or candy.

In about 10 days, you can harvest your natural fertilizer for your garden. For more information on worm tending, go to www.wormdigest.org

Build a Scarecrow Planter

Paint or use stickers on a three-gallon bucket to create your scarecrow's face. To build the body, start with a six- to eight-foot long four by four. Screw on a three-foot two by two for the arms about six inches down from the top of the pole. Invert a five-inch pot onto the top of the pole, and top with a three-gallon bucket screwed into the top of the pole. Sink the pole into the ground about 24 inches. Now fill the bucket with potting soil. Either plant grown grass or sprinkle grass seed, and watch the hair grow. Your scarecrow can wear old clothes and gloves.

Make a Beach

In a corner of your garden, spread sand, pieces of driftwood and shells. Children enjoy the simplicity of the soothing sand and shells. Add a conch shell so they can hear the ocean too!

Grow Your Own Sock Worm

Gather old socks or unmatched pairs. Have the children paint faces on the ends or glue faces on with pieces of felt

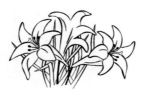

cloth and wiggly eyes. Fill the sock about three-quarters full with potting soil and close off the end with a rubber band or tightly pulled thread. "Water" the worm gently, just to get him damp. Sprinkle on grass seed and let him grow!

Plant a Pizza

Start with a large six- to eight-foot circular plot of turned soil. Mark off triangular plots for each of your six or more pizza parts. Add small logs or rocks around your circle for the pizza crust. Your pizza can be edible or just pretty. If you want an edible pizza garden, plant onions, tomatoes, oregano, peppers, basil and parsley. You will want at least three plants per "slice". Mulch with straw for the cheese! Make sure you harvest your crops, and enjoy a real slice of homemade pizza. If you want to plant a floral pizza, choose flowers that are red, yellow, green and white.

Scented Bundles

Using twelve inch by twelve inch squares or pre-made bandannas, tie up some of the wonderful aromatic herbs you've grown and drop the bundles into drawers, closets or backpacks for a delightful scent. Lavender is particularly great to use, but don't forget mint, cilantro and dill. You can also roll the fabric with the herbs in it to make a bracelet to wear!

Paint Rocks or Birdhouses

Choose smooth stones for the children to paint things such as ladybugs and bees. Place the stones outside in the garden area will also help you determine if the plants need water. Simply turn a stone over that is near any plant, and if

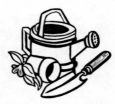

it is damp on the bottom, it does not need watering. If it's dry, it does!

Pre-assembled birdhouses can be purchased at most craft or home supply stores. Do-it-your-self kits for making edible birdfeeders are also available!

Make Plant Markers

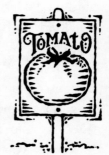

Easy markers made of popsicle sticks and permanent markers work well. Use some imagination and make rock markers, stick ping pong balls on the ends of dowels with silly faces on one side and the plant name on the other. Laminate pictures from gardening magazines on popsicle sticks or dowels.

Fashion a Topiary

Bend a wire coat hanger into the desired shape. Two twisted together can make a butterfly, and one can be fashioned into a heart, a simple circle, a star or a tree. Plant or purchase ivy, and poke your wire into the center of the pot. Gently move your ivy up to attach itself to your form. Give it bright light and water weekly. This is a great project for rainy days or days too hot to go outside. Children still get several sensory feedbacks.

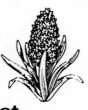

The Sensory Diet

The sensory diet, a term coined by OT Patricia Wilbarger, is a carefully designed, personalized activity schedule that provides the sensory input a person's nervous system needs to stay focused and organized throughout the day.

Proprioception

Proprioceptive input (sensations from joints, muscles and connective tissues that lead to body awareness) can be obtained by lifting, pushing, and pulling heavy objects as well as by engaging in activities that compress (push together) or distract (pull apart) the joints like playing tug-of-war, shovel snow, rake leaves, push heavy objects like firewood in a wheelbarrow, do push-ups against the wall, wear a heavy backpack or pull it on a luggage cart, mow the lawn with a push mower, hopscotch on stones, etc.

Tactile

Tactile input is the sense of touch and includes texture, temperature, pressure, and more. Don't forget that the tactile system includes not only the skin covering your body but also inner skin linings such as inside the mouth.

Auditory

Get out in nature and listen. Go to the beach or sit still and listen to a thunderstorm or windstorm. If you hear birds singing, try to identify what direction a given bird is calling from. Listen to natural sound recordings such as a rainstorm, waves crashing against the beach, or birds in the forest. Sometimes natural sound recordings also feature light instrumentation with flutes, keyboards, etc. These can help create a peaceful, calm environment.

Smell

Explore scents with your child to find the ones that work best to meet your goal (either to calm or to wake up). While everyone has different preferences, lavender, vanilla, and rose are generally calming. Peppermint and lemon are usually invigorating. Let's say your child needs help staying calm and loves lavender. You can use lavender soaps and bath oils to ease bath time, lavender candles or oils in an aromatherapy burner or machine at bedtime, and lavender body lotion.

The garden is a perfect place for children to actively participate in exploring their senses. It is Nature's readymade therapy and can be quickly adapted to include activities for individual's sensory diet. A well balanced garden allows for all senses to be aroused and provides natural opportunities for proprioceptive, calming vestibular and tactile activities. But as children grow, so do gardens and the opportunities available are as numerous as the objects you use to enhance your garden environment.

Proprioceptive Activities

Using bare feet, if the child will allow it, have them dig their toes and feet into the warm ground. Encourage deep pushing into the dirt, pulling the feet out and digging right back in again.

Make mud with fresh dirt and warm (or cool) water. Encourage the activity as if the child were using putty or modeling clay.

Encourage heavy work activities such as pushing a wheelbarrow loaded with dirt or some rocks. Some children just like to move dirt or rocks from one place to another. If your garden has rocks or stones the child can lift, encourage them to turn over the rocks during each visit. You might surprise them now and then with hidden messages taped to the rocks underside! Raking leaves or moving dirt with a child sized rake provides gross motor workout and proprioceptive feedback. Sweeping with a child sized broom can help clean up all the dirt that has been moved during activities, clean the area and provide feedback.

The garden is a natural place to imitate animals that live in the forest. Encourage children to walk like animals, jump like frogs, crawl like an inchworm, etc.

Using a watering can not only provides a sensory experience, it waters the plants and allows for proprioceptive feedback.

Allow children to "wash" the garden's sidewalk, benches, etc. This activity also plays a dual role as you get a clean, fresh garden and you encourage big range of motion and gross motor planning!

Have the child pretend to be garden tools. For example, have the child be the wheelbarrow as it is being pushed through the garden full of dirt and then dumping it on the pretend area to plant in. Next, encourage the child to be a shovel, using his arms to scoop up pretend dirt and get the area ready. Next comes a hoe, jumping up and down making the holes for the seeds. If you desire, continue planting the seeds, covering them with dirt. Then the child can squat all the way down on the ground and pretend to be the sun, slowly coming up, slowly stretching all those muscles, extending their arms to shine on the tender seeds.

Vestibular Activities

Start with taking the child for slow wagon rides through the garden. Get them used to that environment and motion. When a child is ready, take them for rides through the garden and surrounding area in a wheelbarrow. Be sensitive to the child's fear of tipping over since it is on three wheels instead of four. If possible, add a hammock or net swing to the garden environment. This allows children to have the added vestibular activity and experience the calming of the natural environment, and can be used to wind things down after all the activity.

Tactile Activities

Knowledge of the plants in the garden is important. Some plants can have negative affects on skin, however many of them are wonderful, tactile

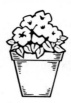

plants to be enjoyed not only with your hands, but gently brushed along a child's arm. Ferns in particular are soft and skin friendly. Lambs ear is another soft, fuzzy plant that almost everyone enjoys touching. Daisys and pussy willow blooms are tactile. Some children may not feel comfortable touching some items. You might consider letting the child decide.

Take a walk through the garden or area. Have children carry a small bag to gather their own items. If working as a group, discuss what each person is picking up. After the walk, sit together and sort into categories of your choice or theirs...long things, living things, heavy things, sticky things, etc.

Encourage exploration to see if you can find seeds (acorns, pods, etc), show children the underside of ferns (spores), what rocks, stones and pebbles can they find? How does each of these things feel? What is the same? What is different?

Move onto plants...Dandelions (even though they are weeds) are so much fun to blow on and stroke for its softness. Ferns are awesome to stroke and explore! Feel the difference in tree leaves...some are pointy, some are round, some are bumpy, some are smooth. Explore the grass. Often exploration starts with just viewing the area and moves to touching with the hands. Encourage exploration with the feet.

Always be aware there are poisonous plants and berries. Make certain you know what the children are exploring!

Explore the outdoors from the bottom to the top. Don't forget tree bark or empty bird's nests.

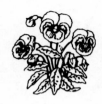

Taste

The obvious things to taste in the garden are foods. Nothing like pulling up a carrot, washing it right there and taking a big bite! You might even find some children will try a new food or texture just because of the change of scenery! Look beyond the fruits and vegetables in the garden and try some herbs. There are varieties of mint (lemon, peppermint, chocolate mint etc) you can try. Don't forget parsley and dill! See if the children will try a piece of (clean) grass. Remember chewing on the tender parts of grass when you were little? Try spinach or cabbage raw…sometimes a child will eat the vegetable in its natural state rather than steamed or cooked. Remember, you are just tasting!

Scent

No one can adequately describe the smell of the outdoors. Try and catch a time when you can smell the rain coming, or just after a rain shower. Can you smell snow? What about the dirt when the sun has been warming it all day? Is there a difference when it is wet? Most of us gravitate toward the scent of the flowers but don't forget the other outdoor elements. Once children become familiar with different scents, they may feel more comfortable with touching or tasting when appropriate. Of course, there is the wonderful scent of mint, lavender, and many flowers. Be mindful that some herbs must be touched or bruised to release its scent.

We are so fortunate that Nature has provided us and our children the perfect environment for learning and growing. For some children, the outdoors is a scary place, for others

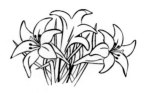

an opportunity to learn and experience new things.

Don't be afraid to just watch what they do naturally...it can be amazing! Children are often telling us what they need and want...we just need to listen.

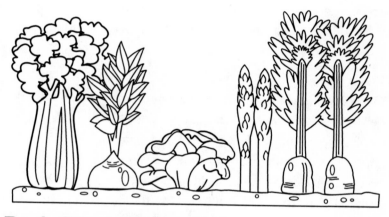

Basic Plant Information

Start with choosing what kind of plants you want in the garden. Annuals are plants that grow for one season or year and then die. Perennials live year after year. Both are fine and grow side by side. You can purchase plants at your local nursery or garden center and you can also buy from mail order catalogs or botanical web sites.

It is usually safe to plant after the last spring frost or before the first frost in the fall. Your local Extension Agency can help with that information if you need it. To plant, dig a hole slightly

larger than the plants root ball. Gently slide the plant out of its container. Using fingers loosen compacted soil and gently fluff out the plants roots. If the plant is extremely root bound use a knife to cut partway into the root ball in several places. Place your plant in the prepared hole, spreading the roots out evenly. Fill the rest of the hole with soil and press it firmly around the plant. Water thoroughly and mulch (for more information about mulching, see the section on Maintenance later in this book). Plants need just a few basic things to thrive: food, water and sunshine.

Watering

The roots of most healthy plants generally grow to a depth of between six and twelve inches, about one-inch of water per week supplied from rainfall or by hand watering should be adequate for healthy plant growth. That inch of watering is best delivered in one long soaking rather than several short ones. The best time to water is early in the morning or the evening when the air is cool and still. Using a rain gauge, which can be purchased at most nurseries, can help you determine how much rain has fallen per week. Keeping the ground moist is important, and adding mulch will help retain the water. Another way to see if the plants need water is to place a smooth stone (about the size of an adult hand) by the plants and leave it there. When the stone is damp, the plant does not need water yet. If the stone is dry, it does!

Food

Composting is an excellent way to add nutrients back into the soil; however, commercial plant fertilizer is also good.

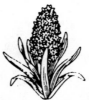

There are two types of fertilizers, organic and chemical. Both work well provided directions on the label are followed. Use a general fertilizer for both plants and vegetables. Most perennials thrive with a spring application of fertilizer (5-10-5 combination). The three numbers stand for Nitrogen, Phosphorous and Potassium respectively. These are the primary nutrients needed by plants in the greatest amounts. Nitrogen encourages leaf and stem development, phosphorous stimulates the root system, and potassium helps plants produce sizeable flowers and fruits.

Sunshine

Plants differ in the amount of sunlight they require. Some do better in full sun, (six to eight hours of direct sun per day) while others need shade. Plants usually need six to eight hours of direct or indirect sun per day. Information is usually available on the tag that comes with a purchased plant but is readily available through books and the Internet. Most plants come with guides that indicate full sun, sun to part shade, or shade and this information will be a great resource in planning and care.

As you're planning your garden, pay attention to water accessibility, drainage, sun exposure, wind and soil composition. That will help in determining what you need to start with and what kind of plants will thrive in your area.

Maintenance

Our goal is to help anyone make a successful garden, but it does take some time. Ideally for a children's sensory garden most of the work is done with the children, but some things may have to be done by adults or parent volunteers. A garden also needs mulch, defined edges, pruning, staking and weeding.

Mulch keeps weeds down, moisture in the soil and helps give garden beds a finished look. There are two types of mulch. Organic and Inorganic. Organic mulches include; pine needles, pine bark, wood chips, leaves, compost, straw, hay, grass clippings and manure. These will break down over time and add nutrients back into the soil. Inorganic mulches include rocks and stone, which only provide weed protection. You can also use landscape fabric (purchased at local nurseries and garden centers) or a one-inch thick layer of newspaper under the mulch to further help keep weeds at bay and hold moisture in the soil. Your mulch is also a part of the sensory affect you are trying to achieve. You can mulch with cedar chips (smell, touch, sight), pine straw (smell, touch), dry grass or leaves. After the holidays, if you can get some Christmas trees shredded, the scent is wonderful, and you have taken care of some discarded trees!

Garden edges are necessary to give you a beginning and end for where the plants are to be and where people can be. Simple additions of edging material can be done with bricks, stones or timber. The areas do not all have to be edged, as you want garden visitors to be able to get close and experience what they see.

Pruning is vital to plant growth and health. Some perennials need to be pinched to encourage fullness and produce more blooms. Simply pinch plant tips with your fingers once or twice during the late spring. One recommendation is to pinch until Mother's Day. Plants that benefit from pinching are mums, asters, phlox and salvias. Children will enjoy pinching; just make sure you give them some guidance!

Deadheading is another activity children will enjoy. After a flower blooms, the bloom should be removed to keep plants pretty and stimulate more blossoms.

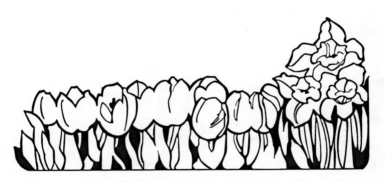

Don't Have a Garden Plot?

Don't let the shortage of ground space prevent you from having a sensory garden. If you have a deck or patio you can still create a sensory garden. Purchase different sized large containers and plant with the plants suggested in this book. Make sure containers have a hole in the bottom for drainage. Use potting soil purchased at a nursery or garden center. And most importantly, water frequently as plants in pots dry out much quicker than those planted in the ground. You may need to water daily in the heat of the summer if there has been no rainfall. Add a water fountain, hang a wind chime, pull up a bench and enjoy.

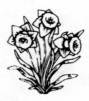

The Four Seasons

Spring

Spring is the time to go to work. Prune, plant and add mulch to the beds. Prune trees and shrubs. Prune bushes such as Beauty Berry and Butterfly Bushes to keep from growing too large. They should be cut back drastically to about one foot tall. Visit local nurseries and garden centers to select your plants and seeds. You can effectively plant, fertilize and water your garden by following the instructions in this book.

Summer

Summer is the time to relax and enjoy what your have created. Sit under the shade of a tree and listen to the rustle of the grass, songs of birds and the trickle of water in a fountain. Smell the gentle fragrance of your summer flowers and feel the coolness of the grass beneath your feet.

Fall

Take advantage of the four seasons to explore how nature changes. School usually starts in the fall, so the area of your garden can be prepped before it gets too cold to have the children outside for long periods of time. They can sit on the ground and dig the dirt, remove any unwanted material, get the area ready for a time of rest or harvest if your garden is all ready established.

While outside, watch the trees change and drop their leaves. The sensational color show Nature puts on cannot be duplicated. Nor can the sound of rustling leaves as they drop through the air to land at our feet or wheelchairs. Now hear the crunch, crunch, crunch as you move through the area!

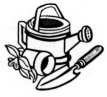

Nature is getting ready to go to sleep for the winter.

You can mulch the leaves to keep the ground covered and they will add nutrients to your soil as it rests and waits for your return in the spring!

Winter

Winter is when planning takes place. You can finalize what you want in your garden. Are you planting seeds or plants or both? Learn about your planting zone and design your plot. Your children can make plant markers (mentioned in Fun Things to do with Kids Chapter), paint pots, work with soil and start seeds. The anticipation helps with the energy you want to capture in the Spring! But don't stay inside, because it is cold! Allow the children to feel the cold earth, to see nature sleeping as most of the trees and bushes in the area are now barren. But there are always evergreens around too! Encourage them to notice what is bare and what is still green and growing.

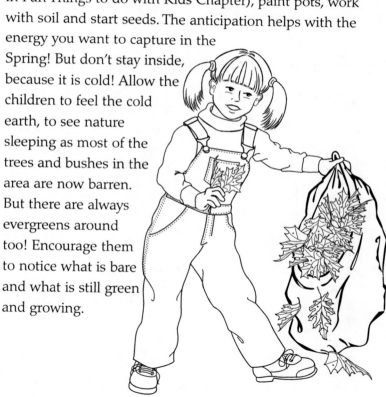

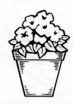

Bringing Your Garden Indoors

Because most schools close for the summer and some areas have harsh winters, you might consider planting a portion of your plants in containers that can be moved inside the classroom. Planters on wheels or in lightweight pots will work both inside and outside. Make sure you have good drainage (whether with a hole in the bottom of the plant and a saucer to catch the water, or small rocks in the planters to create a barrier so the plant is not always wet). Moving the plants inside also can benefit those children who are not comfortable outside but would like to be part of the experience. Containers are readily available at all discount stores, nurseries and even through select supply catalogs.

Plants for the Sensory Garden

Visually Vibrant

Butterfly Bush
Calendula
Elephant Ears
Johnny Jump Ups
Lupine
Marigolds (also keeps bad insects away)
Orange Daisys
Pansies
Sunflowers (Average growth
  is one foot in height a week!)
Violas
Zinnia

Plants and Products for Soothing Sounds

Bamboo Bark*
Chimes
Corn
Fountain Grass
Gravel
Pampas Grass
Pebbles
Water Fountain and Container
Zebra Grass

*(Note: some bamboo spreads very aggressively.)

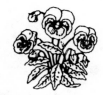

Plants That Feel Fantastic

Bark
Black Eyed Susan
Coneflower
Cosmos
Giant Caladium
Globe Thistle
Horehound

Lambs Ear
Millet (grass)
Pampas Grass
Pussy Willow
Silvermound
Silver Sage
Tansy

Sensational Scents

Alyssum
Chocolate
Citronella Plant
Confederate Jasmine
Curry Plant
Dill
Gardenia
Heather

Honeysuckle
Lavender
Lemon Balm
Lilac
Rosemary
Sage
Sweet Pea

Papery Plants

Globe Amaranth
Money Plant
Sea Oats
Statice
Strawflower

Soft and Silky
Crape Myrtle
Gerbera Daisy
Hibiscus
Peony
Poppy

Fury And Feathery

Astilbe
Celosia
Fennel

Fern
Hare's Tale Grass

Totally Tasty

FOLLOW THE RULE; WHEN IN DOUBT, DO WITHOUT.

Chives
Dandelion Leaves (young)
Hibiscus
Honeysuckle
Nasturtium

Rosemary
Spearmint
Snapdragons
Tulip
Wild Strawberry

Landscape Plans

The following are three simple basic landscape plans. All are handicapped accessible. The plants suggested are common, easy to find, easy to care for plants, and can be purchased at most nurseries, garden centers, or through mail order catalogs. Note most plants purchased through mail order will only be quart size. For larger sizes visit a nursery or garden center.

Landscape Design 1
16' x 16' overall, 3' wide walkway

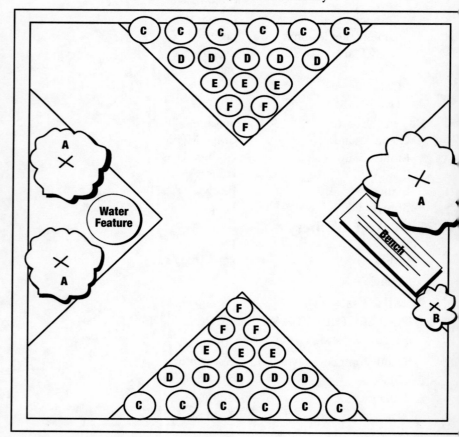

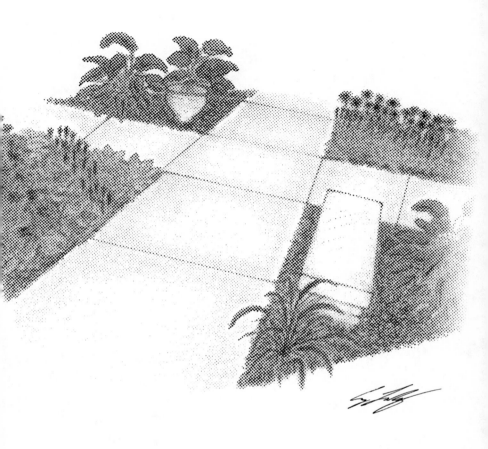

For Design 1 you will need:

A   3, 2 gal. Butterfly Bushes
B   1, 2 gal. Fountain Grass
C   12, 1 gal. Bee Balm
D   10, 1 gal. Yarrow
E   6, 1 gal. Lavender
F   6, 1 gal. Lambs Ear

Landscape Design 2

12' Dia. Outside, 6' Dia. inside, 4' wide walkway

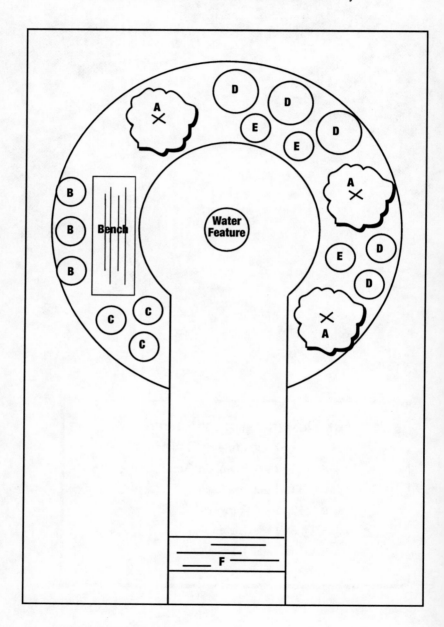

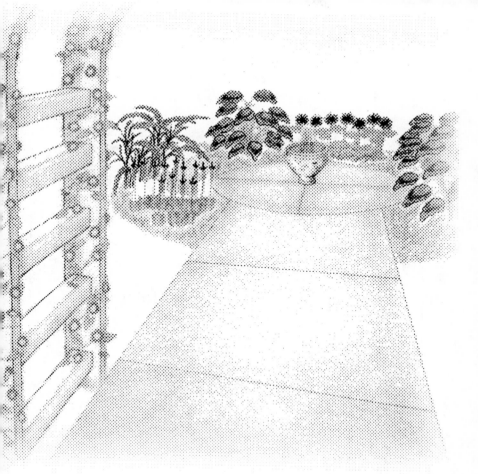

For Design 2 you will need:

- **A** 3, 2 gal. Butterfly Bushes
- **B** 3, 1 gal. Fountain Grass
- **C** 3, 1 gal. Lavender
- **D** 5, 1 gal. Bee Balm
- **E** 3, 1 gal. Yarrow
- **F** 1, pkg. Climbing Morning Glory seeds

Landscape Design 3

10' x 16' overall, 3' x 6' each bed, 4' wide walkways

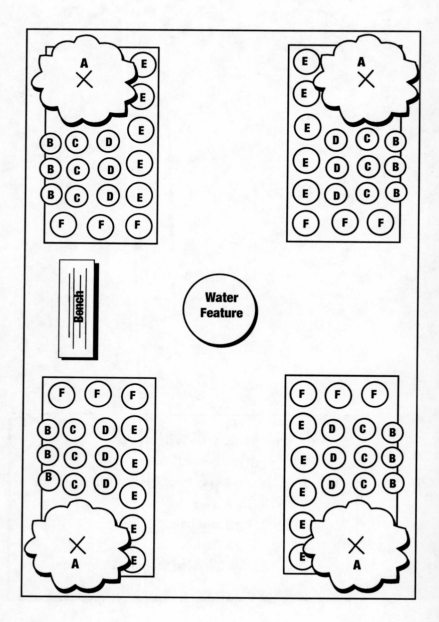

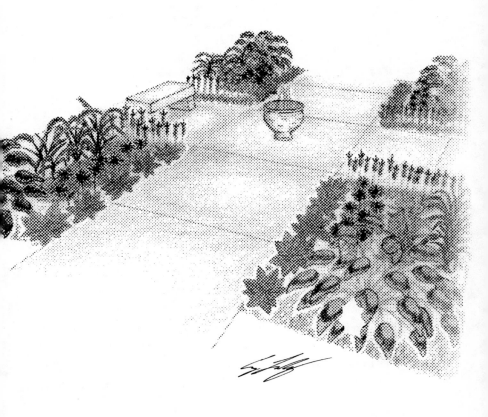

For Design 3 you will need:

A   4, 2 gal. Butterfly Bushes
B   12, 1 gal. Fountain Grass
C   12, 1 gal. Yarrow
D   12, 1 gal Bee Balm
E   20, 1 qrt. Lambs Ear
F   12, 1 gal. Lavender

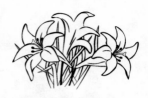

Sensory Garden Assistance

Potential Sources for Grants

National Gardening Association grants of up to $500 for 300 schools ....
....www.garden.org

Grant information available from .... www.kidsgardening.com/grants.asp

Grants and information ....www.herbsociety.org

Childrens Gardening grants ....www.hort.vt.edu/human/Cggrants.html

National Tree Trust funding ....www.nationaltreetrust.org

Agencies

American Association of Botanical Gardens and Arboreta ....www.mobot.org

American Horticultural Society ....www.ahs.org

Keep America Beautiful...www.kab.org

National Arbor Foundation gives 10 tree seedlings for membership ....
....www.arborday.org

National Audubon Society ....www.audubon.org

National Wildlife Federation..www.nwf.org/kids/

Trees for Kids www.realtrees4kids.org

Helpful Websites

Birding information ....www.bestnet.com

Farmers Almanac ....www.almanac.com

Gardening with Kids...www.seedsofknowledge.com

Gardens for Growing People...www.svn.net/growpepl/

Great tips, gardening, ideas, crafts.............................www.oldfashionedliving.com

Info site, kids gardening ideas ....www.mastergardenproducts.com

Kids gardening site, great ideas..www.kidsgardening.com

More gardening with kids ....www.gardenweb.com

Seeds for Kids ....www.for-wild.org/seedmony.htm

Tips, plants and gardening with kids.....................................www.ligardening.com

Wonderful information for kids gardening ....www.bbc.co.uk/gardening
    (Check out Gardening with Children)

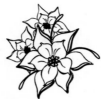

Agencies with Helping Hands

(Don't be afraid to ask....many people are willing to help and fund projects!)

Boy Scouts of America (higher ranking scouts looking for projects for Eagle Rank) They can source the funding, volunteer hours and design. Call your local Boy Scout office for information.

Local 4-H Organization

Local Extension Agency

Local High School (ask for service organizations)

Local PTA

Local Rotary Club

Local Senior Citizens Club

Host a plant shower to get your garden started

Basic Books

Jerry Baker's Old Time Gardening Wisdom by Jerry Baker and Kim Adam Gasier

Jerry Baker's Perfect Perennials by Jerry Baker

Better Homes and Gardens Complete Guide to Flower Gardening by Susan A. Roth

Rodale's Flower Garden Problem Solver by Jeff and Liz Ball

Rodale's Illustrated Encyclopedia of Perennials by Ellen Phillips and C. Colston Burrell

Trowel and Error by Sharon Lovejoy

Notes

Notes

Notes

Printed in the United States
89273LV00002B/1/A

9 780977 184941